# EMERGENCY CARE FOR TRAUMA PATIENTS

## ESSENTIAL EMERGENCY MEDICAL CARE SERVICES

Dr John Paul MD

Dr John Paul MD

Copyright © 2017
Dr John Paul MD

Disclaimer

All the material contained in this book is provided for educational and informational purposes only. No responsibility can be taken for any results or outcomes resulting from the use of this material. While every attempt has been made to provide information that is both accurate and effective, the publisher does not assume any responsibility for the accuracy or use/misuse of this information.

# Contents

_ Transportation of the Trauma Patient

-Extras

# Introduction

Trauma cuts across all national boundaries. Many developing and 3$^{rd}$ world countries have a greater proportion of road traffic accidents and industrial related trauma in a generally younger population.

The management/care of severe multiple injured patients require clear recognition and understanding of treatment priorities and the goal here is to determine during the initial assessment those injuries that are life threatening the patient.

Mortality associated with such

trauma can be reduced by early and effective medical intervention. This manual intends to provide basic knowledge and skills set which is necessary to identify and treat those traumatized patients who require rapid evaluation, quick resuscitation and stabilization of their injuries.

This Manual will particularly highlight the need for early warnings, recognition and timely intervention in life-threatening conditions before it's too late. It provides basic foundation on which doctors, nurses and allied health workers can build knowledge and skills for trauma management with minimal equipment and without advanced and sophisticated technological requirements.

There are several other very successful and well organized trauma courses and manuals available, including the American College of Surgeons ATLS™ course and the EMST Australian course.

These courses are directed to medical personnel in well-equipped hospitals with oxygen; life supports systems, high dependency units, communication and transport etc. and offers a comprehensive training package.

The manual is not a substitute for these courses, but will uses simibasic principles and emphasizes basic trauma care with minimal resources.

# CHAPTER ONE

## THE OBJECTIVES:

At the completion of this course you should:

1. Understand the priorities of trauma management

2. Be able to rapidly and accurately assess trauma patients needs

3. Be able to resuscitate and stabilize trauma patients

4. Know how to organize basic trauma care in your hospital.

## TRAUMA OVERVIEW

Most countries, many developing and $3^{rd}$ world countries experiences an epidemic of trauma, but the most

spectacular increase has been in the developing countries. Proliferation of roads and use of vehicles has led to a rapid increase in injuries and deaths and many peripheral medical facilities find themselves faced with multiple casualties from bus crashes or other disasters. Severe burns are also common in both urban and rural areas.

A number of important differences between high and low-income countries make development of a specifically designed Primary Trauma Care Course beneficial.

# THEY INCLUDE:

- Long travel distance to reach a medical facility and poor infrastructures

- Lack of skilled and trained personnel to operate and service the unit.

- Lengthy time taken for patients to reach and get access proper medical care

- Lack of high-tech equipment and supplies

# CHAPTER TWO

## PREVENTION IS BETTER THAN CURE:

This is by far the most cost effective and safest approach to trauma care and management.

Factors affecting the above includes:-

- Cultural values and ethics

- Personnel

- Power and Political issues

- Financing dilemma

- Training availability.


It's important that the medical

trauma teams make efforts to address the above issues in the prevention of trauma. Much of which this lies beyond the scope of this book, but time will be spent on the course looking at local circumstances and prevention possibilities.

## A-B-C-D-E

The ABCDE survey (Airway, Breathing, Circulation, Disability and Exposure)_The primary' survey, When done correctly should identify life threatening injuries such as:

1. Airway -- for obstruction assessments

2. Breathing – for difficulties plus associated chest injuries assessments

3. Circulation – for Severe hemorrhage either external or internal assessment

4.   Abdominal  injuries

In cases of more than one injured patient then treat patients in order of priority- Triage.

# CHAPTER THREE

## TRIAGE

This is the sorting of patients according to their need for treatment and the resources available. It starts at the scene and continues at the receiving medical facility.

Priority is given to patients most likely to deteriorate clinically and triage takes account of vital signs, prehospital clinical course, mechanism of injury, age and other medical conditions.

A team approach is demanding of personnel and resources.

In trauma centers, teamwork should ensure critically injured patients are evaluated as diagnostic procedures are performed simultaneously, thus reducing the time to treatment.

In smaller institutions, nonhospital settings or with mass casualties, available personnel and resources can rapidly be overwhelmed:

- Triage is done according to the 'ABC' principles below (Airway with cervical spine protection,
  - Breathing, Circulation and hemorrhage control).
- Selection of hospital according to available services, so that trauma patients should be taken to trauma centers.
- **Multiple casualties**. Where the number of patients and severity of injury do not exceed the capacity of the treatment center, life-threatening injuries and

multiple system injuries are treated first.

- **Mass casualties.** When the number of patients and severity of injury do exceed capacity of the treatment center, patients are selected for treatment according to best chance of survival with least expenditure of resources (time, personnel, equipment, supplies).

## PRIMARY SURVEY:

Must be performed in no more than 2–5 minutes.

## Resuscitation and primary survey

For speed and efficacy a logical sequence of assessment to establish treatment priorities must be gone through sequentially although, with good teamwork, some things will be done simultaneously (resuscitation procedures will begin simultaneously with the assessment involved in the primary survey, *ie lifesaving measures are initiated when the problem is identified*). Special account should be taken of children, pregnant women [9] and the elderly [10] as their response to injury is modified. The primary survey is according to:

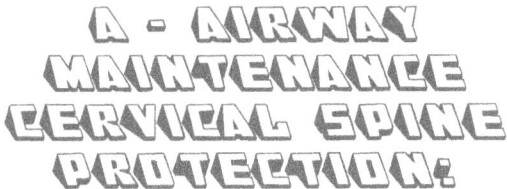

A - AIRWAY MAINTENANCE CERVICAL SPINE PROTECTION:

Are there signs of airway obstruction, foreign bodies, facial, mandibular or laryngeal fractures?

Management may involve secretion control, intubation or surgical airway (e.g. crico-thyroidotomy, emergency tracheostomy).

Establish a clear airway (chin lift or jaw thrust) but protect the cervical spine at all times. If the patient can talk, the airway is likely to be safe; however, remain vigilant and recheck. A nasopharyngeal airway should be used in a conscious patient; or, as a temporary measure, an oropharyngeal airway in an unconscious patient with no gag reflex. Definitive airway should be established if the patient is unable to maintain integrity of airway; mandatory if Glasgow Coma Scale (GCS) less than 8.

Cervical spine protection is critical throughout the airway management process. Movement of the cervical spine could cause spinal injury so movement of the cervical spine should be avoided unless absolutely necessary for maintaining an airway.

The trauma mechanism or history may suggest the likelihood of a cervical spine injury, but always assume there is a spinal injury until proven otherwise, especially in any multisystem trauma or if there is an altered level of consciousness. Inline immobilization and protection of the spine should be maintained and X-rays can be taken once immediately life-threatening conditions have been dealt with.

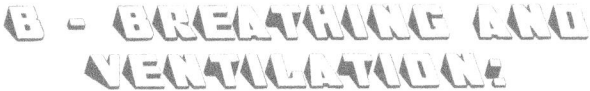

B - BREATHING AND VENTILATION:

Provide high flow oxygen through

rebreathe mask if not intubated and ventilated. Evaluate breathing: lungs, chest wall, and diaphragm. Chest examination with adequate exposure: watch chest movement, auscultate, and percuss to detect lesions acutely impairing ventilation:

Tension pneumothorax- requires needle thoracotomy followed by drainage.

Flail chest - management involves ventilation.

Hemothorax - will usually require intercostal drain insertion.

**Pneumothorax: may require intercostal drain insertion**

**Note:** it can be difficult to tell whether the problem is an airway or ventilation problem. What appears to be an airway problem, leading to intubation and ventilation, may turn out to be a pneumothorax:

or tension pneumothorax which will be exacerbated by intubation and ventilation.

Dr John Paul MD

# CHAPTER FOUR

## C - CIRCULATION WITH HEMORRHAGE CONTROL:

Blood loss is the main preventable cause of death after trauma. To assess blood losses rapidly observe:

Level of consciousness.

Skin color.

Pulse.

Assess circulation, as oxygen supply, airway patency and breathing adequacy are re-checked. If inadequate, the steps to be considered are:

• stop external hemorrhage

- establish 2 wide-bore IV lines (14 or 16 G) preferably
- administer fluid as soon as possible if available.

NB: Bleeding should be assessed and controlled if possible as follows:-

IV access should be achieved with 2 large cannula (size and length of cannula is determinant of flow not vein size) in an upper limb.

Access by cut down or central venous catheterization may be done according to skills available.

At cannula insertion, blood should be taken for crosshatch and baseline investigations.

IV fluids will need to be given rapidly usually as 500 ml to 1 L warmed boluses (10-20 ml/kg in children). Often 2-3 liters in total is necessary, after 40 ml/kg blood is usually needed (O negative, if typed blood is not available).

Ringer's lactate is the preferred initial crystalloid solution.

Direct manual pressure should be used to stem visible bleeding (not tourniquets, except for traumatic amputation, as these cause distal ischemia).

Transparent pneumatic splinting devices may control bleeding and allow visual monitoring; surgery may be necessary if these measures fail to control hemorrhage.

Occult bleeding into the abdominal cavity and around long-bone or pelvic fractures is problematic but should be suspected in a patient not responding to fluid resuscitation.

Remember hypothermia can lead to abnormal blood clotting.

Avoid solutions containing glucose.

Take any specimens you need for laboratory and cross matching.

Urine - Measure urine output as an indicator of circulation reserve. Output should be more than 0.5 ml/kg/hr. Unconscious patients may need a urinary catheter, if they are persistently shocked

**The goal is to restore oxygen delivery to the tissues.**

The usual problem is loss of blood; fluid resuscitation must be a priority.

• Adequate vascular access must be obtained. This requires the insertion of at least two large-
bores cannulas of 14–16 G preferably. Peripheral cut down may be necessary.

• Infusion fluids normal Saline as first line should be warmed to body temperature if possible (e.g. Pre-warm in bucket of warmed water).

Dr John Paul MD

# CHAPTER FIVE

## BLOOD TRANSFUSION

Beware of possible incompatibility, hepatitis B and HIV risks, even amongst patient's own family.

Blood transfusion must be considered when the patient has persistent hemodynamic instability despite fluid (colloid/crystalloid) infusion. If the type specific or cross-matched blood is not available, type O negative packed red blood cells should be used.

Transfusion should, however, be seriously considered if the hemoglobin level is less than 7 g/dl and if the patient is still bleeding.

# I STOP BLEEDING

• **Injuries to the limbs:** Tourniquets do not work. Besides, tourniquets cause reperfusion syndromes and add to the primary injury. The recommended procedure of "pressure dressing" is an ill-defined entity: Severe bleeding from high-energy penetrating injuries and amputation wounds can be controlled by sub-fascial gauze pack placement *plus* manual compression on the proximal artery plus a carefully applied compressive dressing of the entire injured limb.

• **Injuries to the chest:**

The most common source of bleeding is chest wall arteries. Immediate in-field placement of chest tube drain *plus* intermittent suction *plus* efficient analgesia (IV ketamine is the drug of choice) expand.

### • Injuries to the abdomen:

Damage control laparotomy should be done as soon as possible, where fluid resuscitation cannot maintain a systolic BP at 80–90 mm.

DC laparotomy-- The main objective is to pack the bleeding abdominal quadrants using gauze, where after the mid-line incision is temporarily closed within 30 minutes using towel clamps.

This is a resuscitative procedure that should be done under ketamine anesthesia by any trained doctor or nurse at district level.

# 2 VOLUME REPLACEMENT & WARMING'S

## • Replacement is better warm:

Physiological coagulation works best at 38.5°C; Hypothermia in trauma patients is common during prolonged improvised out-door removals – especially in the tropics, prevention of hypothermia is essential. Per oral and IV fluids should have a temperature at 40–42°C

## • Hypotensive Fluid Resuscitation:

In cases where the hemostasis is insecure or not definitive, volumes should be controlled to maintain systolic BP at 80–90 mm during the evacuation.

NB: Response to blood loss differs in:

Elderly - limited ability to increase heart rate; poor correlation between blood loss and blood pressure.

Children - tolerate proportionately large volume loss but then rapidly deteriorate.

Athletes - do not show the same heart rate response to blood loss.

Chronic conditions and medication may affect response and early on in trauma management will not be known about.

# CHAPTER SIX

## COMPLICATIONS:

## SHOCK

Defined as poor organ perfusion and tissue oxygenation. In the trauma patient it is most often due to hypervolemia NB-As a rule loss *of blood is the main cause of shock in trauma patients.*

The diagnosis of shock is based on clinical findings:

Hypotension, tachycardia, tachypnea, as well as hypothermia, pallor, cool extremities, decreased capillary refill, and reduction in urine production. There are different types of shock including:

# HEMORRHAGIC ( HYPOVOLEMIC) SHOCK

Caused by acute loss of blood or fluids. The amount of blood loss after trauma is often poorly assessed and in blunt trauma is usually underestimated. Remember –

Hypovolemic shock is a life-threatening emergency and must be recognized and treated aggressively.

• Femoral shaft fracture   up to 2 liters of blood loss

• Pelvic fracture up to 2 liters of blood loss

• Large volumes of blood loss can

sometimes be hidden in the abdominal and pleural cavity.

## CARDIOGENIC SHOCK:

Due to inadequate cardiac function.

- Myocardial injury, bruising or contusion
- Cardiac tamponade
- Tension pneumothorax
- Penetrating wound of the heart
- Myocardial infarction.

Assessment of the jugular venous pressure is essential in these circumstances and an ECG should be recorded if available.

## NEUROGENIC SHOCK:

Due to the loss of sympathetic tone,

usually resulting from spinal cord injury, with the classical presentation of hypotension without reflex tachycardia or skin vasoconstriction.

## SEPTIC SHOCK:

Rare in the early phase of trauma but is a common cause of late death (via multi-organ failure) in the weeks following injury. It is most commonly seen in penetrating abdominal injury and burns patients.

## D- DISABILITY

Rapid neurological assessment (is patient awake, vocally responsive to pain or unconscious). There is no time to do the Glasgow Coma Scale so an AVPU is ok; system at this stage is clear and quick.

- A - Awake
- V - Verbal response
- P -  Painful response
- U -  Unresponsive

- After A, B and C above, rapid neurological assessment is made to establish:
  - Level of consciousness, using GCS.
  - Pupils: size, symmetry and reaction.
  - Any lateralizing signs.
  - Level of any spinal cord injury (limb movements, spontaneous respiratory effort).
  - Oxygenation, ventilation, perfusion, drugs, alcohol and hypoglycemia may all

also affect the level of consciousness.

Patients need be re-evaluated continuously at regular intervals as deterioration can occur rapidly and often patients can be lucid following a significant head injury before worsening.

Signs such as pupil asymmetry or dilation, impaired or absent light reflexes, hemiplegia/weakness all suggest an expanding intracranial mass or diffuse edema. This requires IV mannitol, ventilation and urgent neurosurgical opinion.

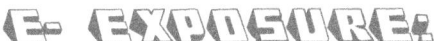

**E- EXPOSURE:**

Undress patient, prevent

hypothermia and look for injury. If the patient is suspected of having a neck or spinal injury, in-line immobilization is important. Clothes may need to be cut off but, after examination, attention to prevention of heat loss with warming devices, warmed blankets etc. Also check blood glucose levels.

# CHAPTER SEVEN

## ADDITIONAL CONSIDERATIONS ( IF RESOURCES ALLOW)

## ECG monitoring:

Help spot dysrhythmias, ischemia, cardiac injury, pulseless electrical activity (PEA) - which may indicate cardiac tamponade - hypervolemia, tension pneumothorax, and extreme hypervolemia.

Hypoxia or hypoperfusion should be suspected if there is bradycardia, aberrant conduction, and premature beats.

Hypothermia produces dysrhythmias.

# URINARY GASTRIC CATHETERS:

- Output of urine can guide fluid replacement (reflects renal perfusion) Adequate output is 0.5-1 ml/kg/hour.

**Note**: prior to catheter insertion urethral injury should be excluded - suspect if there is blood at meatus, pelvic fracture, scrotal blood, Perineal bruising. Per rectum (PR) and genital examination are mandatory prior to catheter insertion.

- Gastric catheters are inserted to reduce aspiration risk. Suction should be applied.

**Note**: care should be taken not to provoke aspiration by triggering gagging.

## OTHER MONITORING:

Monitoring of resuscitation by measuring various important parameters measures adequacy of resuscitation efforts.

Values for various parameters should be obtained soon after the primary survey and reviewed regularly. Important parameters are:

- Pulse rate, [13] blood pressure, ventilator rate, arterial blood gases, body temperature and urinary output.
- Carbon dioxide detectors may identify dislodged endotracheal tubes.

- Pulse oximetry measures oxygenation of hemoglobin calorimetrically (sensor on finger, ear lobe, etc.).

Remember: blood pressure is a poor measure of perfusion.

## Diagnostic procedures

NB: - Do not let these get in the way of the ongoing resuscitation it may be better to deferred it to the secondary survey. Changes to the current ATLS guidelines are currently being looked into. X-rays most likely to guide resuscitation early in the process, especially in blunt trauma, include:

- Chest X-ray.

- Pelvic X-ray. It has been suggested that CT scans may be used in some stable patients.[14]
- Lateral cervical spine X-ray.

Other useful procedures include diagnostic peritoneal lavage (DPL) and abdominal ultrasound to detect occult bleeding.Simultaneous treatment of injuries can occur when more than one life-threatening state exists. It includes:

## SECONDARY SURVEY

This must as a rule begins after the 'ABCDE' of the primary survey, once resuscitation has commenced and the patient is responding with stabilizing vital signs.

This survey is a straight head-to-toe examination with complete history and reassessment of patient's progress, vital signs, and response to treatments.

It requires repeated physical examinations and tends to require further X-ray and laboratory tests. It usually follows the below order.

- **History:**
  - ○ **A** = Allergies
  - ○ **M** = Medication currently used
  - ○ **P** = Past illnesses/Pregnancy
  - ○ **L** = Last meal
  - ○ **E** = Events/Environment related to injury
- **Physical examination:**

Repeat some examinations already undertaken in the primary survey and will be further informed by the progress of the resuscitation. It aims to identify other serious injuries missed in the primary survey, occult bleeding, etc. A review of neurological status including GCS score is also undertaken. Back and spinal injuries are commonly missed and pelvic fractures cause large blood loss which is often underestimated.

## Head to Toe Examination of a Trauma Patient.-

Should take no more than 2-3 minutes

**Neck** - Examine the patient for point tenderness or deformity of the cervical spine. Any tenderness or deformity should be an indication of a possible spine injury. If the patient's C-spine has not been immobilized immobilize now prior to moving on with the rest of the exam. Check to see if the patient is a neck breather, check for tracheal deviation

**Head** - Check the scalp for cuts, bruises, swellings, and other signs of injury. Examine the skull for deformities, depressions, and other signs of injury. Inspect the eyelids/eyes for impaled objects or other injury. Determine pupil size, equality, and reactions to light. Note the color of the inner of the inner surface of the eyelids. Look for blood, clear fluids, or bloody fluids in the nose and ears. Examine the mouth for airway obstructions, blood, and any odd odors.

**Chest** - Examine the chest for cuts, bruises, penetrations, and impaled objects. Check for fractures. Note chest movements a look for equal expansion.

**Abdomen** - Examine the abdomen for cuts bruises, penetrations, and impaled objects. Feel the abdomen for tenderness. Gently press on the abdomen with the palm side of the fingers, noting any areas that are rigid, swollen, or painful. Note if the pain is in one spot or generalized. Check by quadrants and document any problems in a specific quadrant.

**Lower Back** - Feel for point tenderness, deformity, and other signs of injury

**Pelvis** - Feel the pelvis for injuries and possible fractures. After checking the lower back, slide your hands from the small of the back to the lateral wings of the pelvis. Press in and down at the same time noting the presence of pain and/ or deformity

**Genital Region** - Look for wetness caused by incontinence or bleeding or impaled objects. In male patients check for priapism (persistent erection of the penis). This is an important indication of spinal injury

**Lower Extremities** - Examine

for deformities, swellings, bleedings, discolorations, bone protrusions and obvious fractures. Check for a distal pulse. The most useful is the posterior tibial pulse which is felt behind the medial ankle. If a patient is wearing boots and has indications of a crush injury do not remove them. Check the feet for motor function and sensation.

**Upper Extremities** - Examine for deformities, swellings, bleedings, discolorations, bone protrusions and obvious fractures. Check for the radial pulse (wrist). In children check for capillary refill. Check for motor function and strength.

**Rapid Physical Exam** -

## Unresponsive Medical Patient

The rapid physical examination of the unresponsive medical patient is almost the same as the rapid trauma assessment of a trauma patient with a significant mechanism of injury. You will rapidly assess the patient's head, neck, chest, abdomen, pelvis, extremities and exterior.

## Focused Physical Exam - Responsive Medical Patient

The focused physical exam of the responsive medical patient is usually brief. The most important information is obtained through the patient history and the taking of vital signs. Focus the exam on the body part that the patient has the complaint about.

**In a mass casualty situation pay particular attention to following signs and symptoms;**

## Head

- Is headache present
- Are the pupils are the pinpoint, dilated, asymmetrical in size
- Are the conjunctiva injected, draining,
- Does the patient complain of eye pain, photophobia or blurring of vision
- Is salivation, drooling, and/or rhinorrhea present
- Is nasal flaring present
- Note skin color - i.e. is the patient cyanotic
- Note the smell of the patients breath

- Is the patients throat sore, red

## Neck

- Is stridor present
- Are the muscles in the neck "pulling"

## Chest/Lungs

- Note the presence of increased work of breathing i.e. retractions, increased rate
- Note the presence of stridor
- Note the presence of wheezing, rhonchi, rales, decreased breath sounds
- Note the presence of central cyanosis
- Does the patient complain of burning in the chest or chest pain

## Heart/Circulation

- Note the presence of irregular, fast or slow heart rhythms
- Note the presence of diminished or absent peripheral pulse
- Note the presence of prolonged capillary refill in children
- Note the color and temperature of the distal extremities

## Abdomen

- Is the abdomen painful, tense, distended or rigid?
- Does the patient have cramping, vomiting or diarrhea

## Pelvis

- Check for incontinence of urine or feces

## Neurological

- What is the patient's mental status? Is he (she) seizing?
  - Is the patient dizzy?
  - Did syncope occur?
- Was there sudden collapse
- Does he (she) have muscle twitching?

## Skin

- Is the skin painful, burning numb or tingly
  - Is the skin erythematous
  - Are there vesicles, bullae
    - Is there necrosis

Beware:

-Burns have high fluid requirements, inhalation injury.

- Cold injury needs continuous resuscitation until rewarmed.

- Voltage electrical injuries tend to hide extensive muscle injury.

## Additional considerations to secondary survey

Other range of further diagnostic tests and procedures may be required after the secondary survey. These may include CT scans, ultrasound investigations; contrast X-rays, angiography, bronchoscopy, esophageal ultrasound, etc. If this are available

## Definitive care

Choosing where care should continue can be challenging in the tropics especially where resources are scarce, good medical facility plus trained persons are either not available or in short supply, but however most appropriately will depend on results of the primary and secondary surveys and knowledge of the facilities available to receive the patient.

The closest appropriate facility should be "always" be chosen.

## Remember:

- Keep meticulous records at all times for all entries, etc. Teamwork with timekeeping and recording of accurate clinical measurements, and observations can prove to be more than valuable.
- A nursing staff can be charged to accurately record and collate patient care information.
- Consent for treatment is not always possible with lifesaving treatment and consent may have

to be done later when capacity can be determined and evidence may be required in injuries caused by criminal activities.

## REMEMBER

REGULAR TRAINING in resuscitation by the whole practice team is PRICELESS.